FAT

TO

FABULOUS

By Roman Iver

Copyright © 2016

TABLE OF CONTENTS

Chapter I 1

INTRODUCTION 1

Which is More Important, Diet Or Exercise?..2

Preventing Being Overweight is Easier than Losing Weight at Any Age..............2

Chapter II 5

Health Benefits of Weight Loss..5

Rev Up Your Metabolism All Day That Helps Your Body Maintain a Healthy Weight 6

My Friends Are Happy That the Diet Plan I'm Following is Working For Them Too..7

How Do I Decide How Much I Should Weigh? 8

The table below will tell you whether you are underweight, ideal, or overweight 9

A Diet Can Be Healthy But Can Make You Gain Weight Because of Diet Mistakes 9

Reasons Why Your TV is Making You Fat..11

Can You Believe A Diet Plan Can Also Help You Gain Weight? 13

Diet and Diabetes: The Diabetes Meal Plan and Glycemic Index 13

Glycemic Index table...14

Do You Know Why Japanese People Don't Get That Fat? 15

Chapter III **17**

You Know About Physical Strength. Do You Know What Mental Strength Is and Its Importance? 17

Science of Developing Mental Toughness in Life 17

Myths about Mental Strength 19

Reshape Your Mind: 7 Healthy Foods to Take in to Reshape It 22

What Celebrities Say About Mental Illness? 22

Chapter IV **25**

Body Types: Ectomorph, Mesomorph, and Endomorph 25

Body-type Specific Foods 26

Summary 29

Chapter I

INTRODUCTION

Are you clueless about how much you should weigh? Do you need help overcoming obesity? Do you find yourself unable to follow a strict diet plan?

This book will answer all your questions. From this book, you will find out whether your weight is ideal, or if you are under or over the ideal weight. You will also learn the effective techniques to lose, maintain, or gain weight.

It covers the most important objective, "how to lose weight through an effective diet plan." This book also explains the dos and don'ts while you are on a diet.

There is a lecture exclusively for patients with diabetes. It talks about a result-oriented diabetes meal plan. Also, learn about Glycemic Index, a guide to control blood sugar. Know about fast releasing and slow releasing carbs.

Because of our busy schedules and mood changes, we may not be able to stick to a diet plan. Learn about mental strength or mental toughness that helps you do anything with focus. It mentions some myths you should believe to stay focused on your goal.

This book also explains the different body types you know: Ectomorph, Endomorph, and Mesomorph. It also mentions the recommended body-specific foods.

Webster's dictionary defines diet as "to eat less food or to eat only particular kinds of food in order to lose weight: to be on a diet."

This book is written to create awareness about the importance of a balanced diet, exercise, and healthy lifestyle.

Which is More Important, Diet Or Exercise?

An appropriate diet and exercise routine at regular intervals are important for healthy living. However, even without exercise, you probably can have a fairly healthy body as long as your diet is packed with healthy nutrients.

If you are of the opinion that you can feast upon whatever you wish so long as you exercise, then you are mistaken. Also, if your diet is unhealthy, no matter what type of exercise you do, you'll neither stay healthy nor become muscular.

Eat a balanced diet
It's important to include all the macronutrients or the nutrients that give your body calories or energy in your meal. The macronutrients include proteins, carbohydrates, vitamins, minerals, and fat. Not to mention, you should absorb plenty of water.

Preventing Being Overweight is Easier than Losing Weight at Any Age

Overweight and obesity is a sophisticated problem – a world problem. On one hand, they are caused because of genetic make-up, and on the other hand, it is a consequence of modernization of lifestyle and technological advancements – a change from walking to riding, from playing outdoors to indoor games, and from eating healthy foods to fattening fast foods. Also, because of our advanced lifestyles, we have become less active than before.

Fattening fast foods, junk foods, and very little or no exercise are to be blamed according to experts for becoming overweight or obese. Eating more calories than our body burns might lead to obesity.

According to research, about 60% of adult Americans are overweight, and of this, over 30% are obese. In spite of the promotions of healthy diets and physical activities by the media and a huddle of educational campaigns, obesity is still prevailing in the United States. In fact, it has doubled over the last few decades.

Obesity increases the risk of many other health problems including heart diseases, stroke, certain cancers, and diabetes. These diseases can affect a person's quality of life and reduce life expectancy. Hence, it is considered an epidemic.

Adding weight can be avoided by zoning in on healthy eating habits and regular physical activities. It is easier to prevent being overweight or obese than dropping pounds at any age. Timely exercise is the key to attaining an ideal weight and better physique.

You can find out whether you are overweight or obese according to your height by referring to: The table below will tell you whether you are underweight, ideal, or overweight

Another way to find it is with the help of the Body Mass Index (BMI), a measure of fat. BMI is calculated using a formula involving height and weight of your body.

The image below gives you the formula to calculate BMI. However, if you don't want to break your head with the formula. Use the BMI Online Calculator and compare your score with the table below:

Prevent being overweight or obese by adopting the following:

- Healthy eating habits
- Eat more fruits, veggies, nuts and seeds, whole grains etc.,
- Exercise for at least half an hour
- Cut back on fatty and sugary foods.

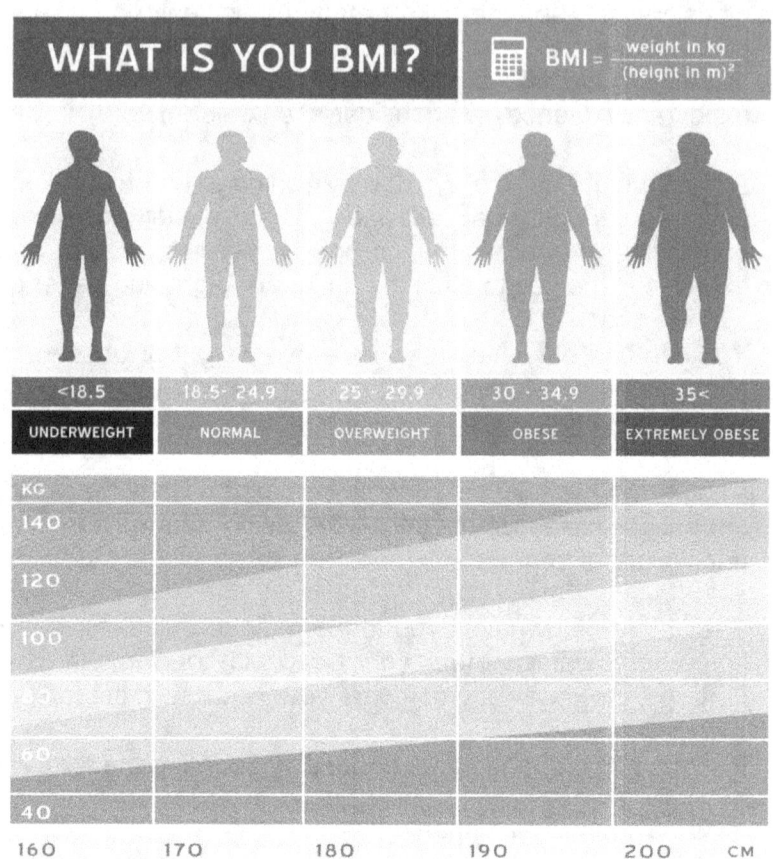

WHAT IS YOU BMI?

$$BMI = \frac{weight\ in\ kg}{(height\ in\ m)^2}$$

<18.5	18.5- 24.9	25 - 29.9	30 - 34.9	35<
UNDERWEIGHT	NORMAL	OVERWEIGHT	OBESE	EXTREMELY OBESE

KG

140

120

100

80

60

40

160   170   180   190   200   CM

Chapter II

Health Benefits of Weight Loss

If you're grossly fat, losing a few pounds can reduce the risk of certain serious health issues. Most people who are obese can achieve health benefits by losing about 5 – 10 % of their body weight.

Refer to the table under the subtitle, "How do I decide how much I should weigh?" that will tell you if you are overweight, and if you are, how much weight you should aim to lose. Here are the benefits you enjoy after losing weight:

Breathe easily, prevent snoring, and improve sleep.
Obese people are likely to develop fatty tissues around the neck, partially blocking the air movement, resulting in snoring. Snoring is likely a symptom of Sleep Apnea, a life threatening condition. Losing a few pounds helps thin down these soft tissues and reduce snoring.

Keep chronic diseases from happening: An A1 Diet Plan can help us stay away from longstanding diseases as we age. These chronic diseases include cardiovascular diseases, some cancers and arthritis.

Weight Joint Pain
Most people who are obese have a common joint disorder known as osteoarthritis that causes the bone and cartilage to wear away. Consequently, the joints become bloated and tender, and mobility becomes exceedingly painful.

In obese people, there is an increase in the load placed on the joints – knees and hips. Even a loss of 5% of the total body weight reduces the stress on these joints and relieves you from pain. By losing 5 kg, you reduce the force of about 15 to 30 kg on the knees.

Prevent Type 2 Diabetes
Type 2 Diabetes or T2D or High Blood Glucose occurs when your body ceases to produce the adequate amount of insulin, or the produced insulin does not work properly.

We know that insulin helps control blood glucose levels. Obesity increases the risk factors of T2D since it causes difficulty for cells to react to the insulin hormones.

By losing weight, you can prevent the development of diabetes from prediabetes. A weight loss of 5 to 10%, coupled with moderate physical activities such as brisk walking can help you avoid T2D.

Psychological benefits

Losing weight not only offers several health benefits, but also enhances body image, self-esteem, and quality of life. According to studies, losing weight tremendously boosts confidence, reduces depression, and enhances the quality of life. You can do any job relatively easily.

Rev Up Your Metabolism All Day That Helps Your Body Maintain a Healthy Weight

The classical definition of metabolism is the overall biochemical process that occurs in our body, or for that matter, any living organisms. Simply put, it's the number of calories we burn every day to release energy.

Metabolism keeps the cells and living beings alive by giving them the essential energy to carry on. They also need energy to grow and reproduce. Metabolism is a process that has to be carried out to sustain life. Without it, living organisms will just die. Living organisms get energy through food and sunlight. Any defects in metabolism can result in health problems. For example, when the body fails to metabolize blood sugar properly, it may result in chronic diseases like diabetes.

A major portion of the calories is used up for functions carried out throughout the day in your body such as breathing and circulation. Another significant portion is burnt by the brain, liver, heart, kidneys, and the digestive system. The physical activities you perform burn about 25% of the calories.

You need to know how your body functions since this knowledge helps you choose the appropriate diet and enhance the benefits you can enjoy from it.

My Friends Are Happy That the Diet Plan I'm Following is Working For Them Too

Losing weight is on the top of my list like many others in the United States as I'm concerned about my bulging waistline. I was longing for a diet plan that really works and is safe. I tried several diet plans to lose weight, but most of them make me hungry and I give up dieting.

Finally, a dietician who is also my dad's friend said, "Whether you want to lose weight or maintain your current weight, you need to stick to a good diet plan." He also gave me a few other tips, and from then on, I just stick to 3 meals and a snack each day. This workout plan has assured me a weight loss of nearly 15 pounds by the end of 5 weeks and I have been seeing some differences already. I recommended this diet plan to a few of my friends, and they are happy too. Remember! You've got to have a strong will because if you don't, you'll call it a day because of hunger.

This is what the plan will do.

1. Make you feel full and lessen your appetite significantly
2. Help you quickly drop pounds
3. Speed up your metabolism

Reduce the amount of sugars and starches in your diet
Insulin is a hormone that stores fat in your body and food rich in sugars and starches (carbs) accelerate the secretion of this hormone. When you cut back on insulin, fat easily gets out. That's to say your body starts burning fat. One more use of reducing insulin is that excess sodium and water releases from your kidneys and in turn, leaves your body. As a result, surplus bloat and water weight is reduced.

With this style of eating, you can burn body fat as well as reduce water weight significantly. You'll not be surprised to drop nearly 10 pounds in the first week.

Each of your meals should have carbs, vegetables, a source of protein, and a source of fat. Examples of protein sources are meats such as chicken and beef, and fat sources include x, y, and z.

Fat sources are foods like eggs (pasteurized or Omega-3 enriched). Your meals should also include fish and seafood – salmon, shrimps, lobsters, etc.

Proteins lift the metabolism by nearly 100 calories a day. Diets rich in proteins reduce the craving for midnight or late night snacking. They make you feel full so that you automatically consume fewer calories.

Low carb veggies include, broccoli, spinach, cauliflower, lettuce, cabbage, kale, Swiss chard, celery, cucumber, and Brussels sprouts.

Rule of thumb: construct your everyday meal out of a source containing proteins, fat and low carb vegetables.

Include physical activities
Perform some warm up exercises, stretching exercises, and lifting weight without going to the gym, although going to a gym is an effective option (at least 3 to 4 times a week). The best part about the gym is the trainer can offer you some valuable advice frequently.

In some cases, metabolism slows down, which is a side effect of losing weight. Lifting weight prevents this and burns a few calories.

Alternatives to lifting weight are running, jogging, swimming, or simply walking.

How Do I Decide How Much I Should Weigh?

This is the most common question that the majority of health conscious people have. To decide what your ideal body weight should be, you must keep in mind a number of factors - age, sex, height, and bone density.
It is worth remembering that your ideal body weight is entirely different from another person. So, comparing yourself with others may not work.

The table below will tell you whether you are underweight, ideal, or overweight

WOMEN				MEN			
Height Ft. In.	Frame Size Small	Med.	Large	Height Ft. In.	Frame Size Small	Med.	Large
4'10"	102-111	109-121	118-131	5'2"	128-134	131-141	138-150
4'11"	103-113	111-123	120-134	5'3"	130-136	133-143	140-153
5'0"	104-115	113-126	122-137	5'4"	132-138	135-145	142-156
5'1"	106-118	115-129	125-140	5'5"	134-140	137-148	144-160
5'2"	108-121	118-132	128-143	5'6"	136-142	139-151	146-164
5'3"	111-124	121-135	131-147	5'7"	138-145	142-154	149-160
5'4"	114-127	124-138	134-151	5'8"	140-148	145-157	152-172
5'5"	117-130	127-141	137-155	5'9"	142-151	156-160	155-176
5'6"	120-133	130-144	140-159	5'10"	144-154	151-163	158-180
5'7"	123-136	133-144	143-163	5'11"	146-157	154-158	161-184
5'8"	126-139	136-150	146-167	6'0"	149-150	157-170	164-188
5'9"	129-142	139-153	149-170	6'1"	152-164	160-174	168-192
5'10"	132-145	142-156	152-173	6'2"	155-168	163-178	172-197
5'11"	135-148	145-159	155-176	6'3"	158-172	167-182	176-202
6'0"	138-151	148-162	158-176	6'4"	162-176	171-187	181-207

A Diet Can Be Healthy But Can Make You Gain Weight Because of Diet Mistakes

Many people aren't happy because they are gaining weight in spite of following a diet plan. According to experts, you might be devouring more calories than you ponder when you are dieting. Possibly some eating mistakes are to be blamed. Below are a few casual mistakes people make while dieting.

Gobbling food down in a few minutes
You aren't on America's "Nathan's hot dog contest," to finish your food in record period. Remember! You're on a diet. Our busy work life has forced us to practice the habit of eating quickly. We need to change this. We must adopt a leisurely style eating so as to taste and enjoy every bit and bite of the food. This way, you can keep from overeating.

Skipping meals, especially breakfast

The fact that you can prevent the calories from sneaking into your body by skipping meals is a myth. A recent study says, people who skipped breakfast weighed more than those who didn't. In actual fact, many people who eat less than three meals a day cram down more calories.

Begin with a healthy breakfast: have 3 meals a day.

Feeding yourself too much liquid calories

According to recent research, Americans consume about 21% of calories in the form of calorie-loaded beverages including juices, smoothies, sodas, and alcohol. Beverages fulfill your thirst and don't affect your hunger. Thus, by drinking beverages, you don't compensate by eating less. Choose from low calorie beverages such as water, vegetable juices, and small portions of pure fruit juices.

Stuffing down large portions of meals

Restaurants serve large portions of enticing, mouth-watering cuisines to impress us, and we think this is of standard size so we adopt the same measure at home.

The best way to ensure you eat the correct portions of food is to use measuring cups to serve food for yourself, and regularize it.

Also, calories can add up by mindless eating - unknowingly emptying the snacks from a bag while watching TV.

Including unhealthy food supplements

Besides eating larger portions of food, we usually top them up with high fat, high calorie toppings like cheese, bacon, and honey.

Calories can accumulate quickly and you won't even realize it. They can be removed as quickly too. Getting acquainted with the common diet mistakes and the ways calories enter your body day in and day out, amount to real weight loss.

Reasons Why Your TV is Making You Fat

Computers, Televisions, and gadgets such as video games, smartphones, and tabs are to be blamed for keeping us desk-bound and attached to these, but according to researchers, the Television is the biggest culprit that is accountable for weight gain that increases the risk of certain diseases related to obesity. Consequently, it reduces the viewer's life expectancy. Here are the following reasons why TV can make you fat:

Your hands are free for Munching
Indulging in video games or computers is not associated with weight gain since your hands are busy typing or texting. On the other hand, while watching Television, your hands are freed and are tempted to grab your favorite snacks. While it is virtually impossible to shun TV-watching entirely, being aware of the risk of being overweight can control the amount you watch.

It Makes You Choose the Wrong Snacks
While watching Television, your hands are tempted to the snacks nearby without bothering whether they are healthy or not. According to a study, people who are attached to TV have a poorer understanding of nutrition.

It's a Food Peddler
Sometimes, while watching TV, even when you are not hungry, you tend to grab some deep-fried snack and slide into a chair to continue watching TV. After it's over, you drive to the bakery close by to buy some sweets. The munchies shown in TV commercials are more often than not unhealthy. According to a study by the University of Liverpool, people who watched TV commercials for junk foods mostly ordered sugary and high-fat foods than those who watched commercials for non-consumable foods, or nature programs.

It Obstructs Sleep
Having Televisions in the bedrooms poses a high risk, according to researches. Staring at the TV screen for a long time can interrupt sleep. About 70% of adolescents have TVs in their bedrooms. Also, children who rested in bedrooms having TVs gained nearly one extra pound each year. A simple way of restricting your kid's Television time is to move the TV out of the bedroom.

Shift Your Exercise Equipment Near the Television
Moving your exercising equipment in front of the TV helps you exercise for a long time without boredom. You can run on a treadmill, do some weightlifting, or any other activity.

Exercises Without Exercising Equipment
You don't have any exercising equipment? Don't worry. Perform some free exercises that give work for all your body parts. Here are some free exercises that you can perform while watching TV:

Pushups
Pushups are the best exercises that a newbie to fitness will be able to do. If you are a beginner to fitness, you can do pushups in the commercial breaks, say, about 10 pushups. After you become proficient, try as many pushups as you can in a half an hour program.

Stretching Exercises
Stretching is a good exercise. Follow some full-body stretching exercises whether you are new to fitness or an advanced exerciser. Do a warm up before stretching. Keep in mind not to stretch to the point of pain. Stretching exercises that gives work to every part from head to toe include Neck Stretch, Hamstring Stretch, Quad Stretch, Chest and Biceps Stretch, Standing Triceps Stretch, Back Stretch, and Hip and Gluteal Stretch.

Squat Exercise
Squats are perfect for building your lower body, especially the thighs and buttocks. It also helps you train your core muscles. Squats can be done anywhere as you use just your own body weight. It improves blood circulation, posture, and digestion.

Also, do some free exercises for a Well-shaped upper body and lower Abs.

Can You Believe A Diet Plan Can Also Help You Gain Weight?

When someone says, "I'm on a diet," we assume that they are trying to flaunt a flat stomach. There can be the other reasons too – to gain weight.

People may be thin because of two reasons - heredity or a medical condition. They struggle to add pounds as much as people struggle to subtract pounds. In the quest of gaining weight, it is imperative that you choose the appropriate foods instead of simply stuffing in calories so you can gain weight in a healthy way.

Acquire 3000 calories a day through 3 meals of 750 calories each and 3 snacks of 250 calories each. Include plenty of fruits, vegetables, proteins, and fats at every meal. Eat foods rich in nutrients solid in calories such as nuts and seeds, vegetable oils, almonds, chocolate, dried fruits, avocado, whole grains, oily fish, meat, milk, dairy, and eggs.

Diet and Diabetes: The Diabetes Meal Plan and Glycemic Index

A diabetes meal plan is a guru that tells you the types of food and quantity you can pick at any meal and munching times. A good meal should be a good fit to your plans and eating habits. An appropriate meal plan can help you control your blood sugar, blood pressure (BP), and cholesterol figures. It can also help you track your weight. Whether there is a need for you to take pounds off, or maintain your current weight, your meal plan designed exclusively for you can help.

What is Glycemic Index?
The Glycemic Index or Gycaemic Index or simply GI is a comparatively new way of analyzing foods. It is basically a number that indicates how Co^2 Carbon dioxide affects blood glucose levels.

The GI diet centers on carbs because eating carbs results in a steadier rise in blood sugar. Not to mention, the fiber foods in the carbs help you feel full for longer and more fulfilling. Adopting a low

Glycemic Index diet might help you stay away from conditions such as Diabetes Mellitus and Cardiac diseases.

Also, according to a study, people on a low Glycemic Index diet lost more fat when compared to the ones on a high GI diet with an equal amount of calories.

Glycemic Index can be sometimes mystifying. A food low on the GI may not be healthy and likewise, a food ranked high on it may be nutritious. The GI diet is not a weight shedding diet. Instead, it recommends carbs for diabetes patients who depend on them to control their blood sugar.

Glycemic Index table

Low GI Foods (56-69)	Medium GI Foods (70 or higher)	High GI Foods 55 or lower
Egg and bacon	White rice	Oat meals
Omelet	White bread	Peanuts
Leftovers from previous night's dinner	Pretzels	Peas
Coffee and cream	White bagels	Carrots
Boiled egg with Mayonnaise/butter	White baked potatoes	Kidney beans
Avocado	Crackers	Hummus
Salmon	Sugar sweetened beverages	Skimmed milk
Sour cream	Pizza	Grains
Cheese and butter	Hamburger bun	Pasta
Sandwich on Oopsie bread	Potato	Cereals
High fat yogurt with nuts and seeds		
A piece of brick cheese with some ham/salami		

Do You Know Why Japanese People Don't Get That Fat?

According to a survey conducted by the University of Pennsylvania in 2008, Japan or Nippon is one of the countries that has a very low amount of overweight or obese people in the world, in spite of the presence of thousands of McDonald's outlets. The best part about Japan is the average life expectancy here is one of the longest in the world –86 years for women and 79 years for men as against 80 years and 75 years respectively for Americans. They are among the healthiest people in the world.

Snacking in this country is popular and convenient too. Most urban locations have a number of fast food stalls and restaurants having all types of alluring, ready-to-eat foods that make you fat. The snack industry has been aggressively competitive for decades and people are getting more and more worried about unhealthy fast foods.

This does not mean there are absolutely no overweight or obese people in the country. People in Japan are captivated with foods like their counterparts in America and the United Kingdom. Every now and then, a new interesting diet arrives on the streets.

Most food websites in Japan tirelessly talk about healthy diets and weight loss schemes.

Japanese people have been slim, and it is believed that they'll continue to be slim for a while. Here are a few reasons that back this:

Smaller Meal Portions
The main reason why Japanese people are thin, at least, what Americans who have ballooned to crazy proportions feel (Japanese people aren't that thin in reality), is that they eat real food - homemade; they still cook themselves.

The next reason, most Japanese folks skip lunch; only water (plenty) and green tea might pass their lips at times.

Most importantly, in spite of the unforeseen trends showcasing sizable foods such as Mega burgers, Big Mac sandwiches, and Egg

McMuffins by chain of fast food restaurants like McDonald's, the average size of the meal portion is much smaller than that of the US.

Authentic Japanese Cuisine
Japanese people pride themselves on the quality of their traditional cuisines. They analyze and passionately discuss food.

Their food is mostly based on seafood.

Japanese foods have become more popular and appreciated all over the globe in recent years.

The traditional Japanese cuisine is totally healthy, being considerably squatty in fat and rich in macronutrients, especially carbs, and proteins. The main protein sources include fish, beef, quinoa, peanut butter, oats, avocado, peas, chickpeas, edamame, and beetroot. Connoisseurs of food recommend you to take pleasure in eating the raw fish while you're consuming in the process. In fact, fish is a much more pronounced food on their plates usually. Japanese foods are considered healthier than American foods. The average calorie intake by Japanese people is about 2700 calories per day, about 1000 less than the calorie intake by Americans.

Natural exercise
More often than not, people living in Japan, particularly in the urban and suburban areas move a lot. Most of the people commute by public transportation instead of their personal cars. They use cars only for long distances. This way, the Japanese people get more exercise eliminating the need to go to a gym although there are thousands of them. More movement complements their eating habits. The Japanese exercise more than the Americans.

Chapter III

Mental Strength

You Know About Physical Strength. Do You Know What Mental Strength Is and Its Importance?

Most people spend a lot of time talking and discussing physical strength. Newsstands are often filled with magazines that always talk about weightlifting and fitness. Workout videos account for about 300 USD per year, and TV commercials are dominated by the latest diet and weight loss supplement trends.

Mental strength is interpreted in different ways. However, the general and the most accepted one is a state of mind, mystique in action, and possessing a positive attitude. It is being calm and focused on your ambition and goal in the midst of hindrances and troubles. It is the quality of being mentally strong - boldly admitting your mistakes.

We will not be able to achieve any goals without mental strength. We can reach our full potential in life by building our mental strength. It is the key to achieve our physical fitness goals and brimming potential in the love of our lives. Eating correctly and exercising regularly is a battle physically as well as mentally. If you can achieve this, you'll be able to convince yourself that nothing is impossible. This holds well both for dieting and exercising. While dieting, you might get tempted to go out to eat, or to order a light meal while your friend orders something. The nucleus to strictly follow a diet plan are to stand focused, have control and authority, and be extra cautious so as to prevent yourself from returning to your old habits.

Science of Developing Mental Toughness in Life

Some people become great entrepreneurs, leaders, sports personalities, or acclaimed filmmakers, while others fail.

Why this difference?

There is more than just saying things like, "He is the smartest business strategist," "He is the footballer with the greatest stamina," and so on. That is to say, just talent or intelligence are not the key to success as you might be thinking. They account for only 30% of your achievement. A greater effect than talent and intelligence is 'Mental Toughness.'

Mental toughness, "Will, or "Grit" as one calls it plays a pivotal role for achieving your goals in anything - health, business, or life. It is the ability to remain focused and resolved in spite of the circumstances.

Here are some of the basic steps for developing a new habit.

Building mental toughness is as good as building your body and muscles in gym. This mental exercise will help you focus and be successful. Here are the factors that denote mental toughness:

Self-motivation: The root of mental toughness
The deep-rooted philosophy of mental toughness is motivation. According to sports psychologists, people who are considered mentally tough display innate motivation. A study that was presented in psychology defines mental toughness as the craving for self-determination. Mentally tough people are generally self-motivators and self-starters. They just need encouragement here and there.

Build Your Personal Identity
Your appearances, thoughts and feelings, daydreams and fantasies, make you standout in a crowd. Take good care of your looks since it is a part of your identity. Engage yourself in effective methods to enhance your appearance as a sense of esthetics is necessary for an amusing lifestyle. Your style of talking, body language, and facial expressions together reflect your personality.

Reinvent Your Social identity
Your name, nationality or locality, and religion are components of your social identity. Some people identify themselves by the job they do. Factors such as race, ethnicity, and religious beliefs tell who you are.

Myths about Mental Strength

In spite of the significance of mental strength, not many are acquainted with the concept. There are a lot of misconceptions about the big idea of mental strength. Believe these 5 myths about Mental Strength to prevent the hindrances to interfere in your quest to do something.

Believe these 7 Myths about Mental Strength That Keep You from Focusing on Your Goal

Myth #1: There are two kinds of people: Mentally strong and mentally weak.

Nugget of truth: the idea according to most people that one can be either mentally strong or weak is still a prevalent misconception. The fact of the matter is; we all possess mental strength to some degree. Also, we all have the ability to become mentally stronger.

Building your mental strength is more like building your physique. To build physical muscle, you'll need to develop healthy habits – like eating healthy foods, and going to the gym. You also need to banish unhealthy practices – like eating unhealthy fast foods.

To build mental strength, you'll need to follow some healthy habits:

   a. **Expressing gratitude**
   b. **Get rid of the "give up" attitude after your first attempt**
   c. **Use your mental power intelligently**

Myth #2: Mentally strong people inherited mental strength

Nugget of truth: Mentally strong people aren't born with mental strength, or no one has the impotence to develop emotional, cognitive, and behavioral skills.
A few of them could be different facets of genetic-makeup – the way of thinking, feeling, and behaving. We have to attain it by practice and hard work, and the good news is, it can be learned like any other skill.

Myth #3: Mentally strong people aren't sentimental and friendly

Nugget of truth: Mentally strong people are not robots. Everyone experiences emotions, and mentally strong people are no exception. They know how their emotions play a role in leveraging their thoughts and actions. They have the ability to attain mental toughness that help them achieve their missions without any compromise. They don't allow their emotions to interfere in the process.

Myth #4: Mentally strong people think positively all the time

Nugget of truth: Optimism is a big self-motivator, but having a positive attitude all the time without weighing the circumstances does not sound pragmatic. They manage challenges; consider what is possible and what is not, by holding a positive approach.
Mentally strong people don't start anticipating big things to occur. Nor do they always have happy thoughts. Instead, they are realistic and rational. They try to develop mental strength that increases the ability to assess their thoughts.

Myth #5: Mentally strong people are devoid of mental health issues

Nugget of truth: This is not true. Even mentally strong people have spent days in melancholy and fought mental health issues. They endure pain, depression, and mental health problems, and build mental strength. Mentally strong people train themselves to mull over rationally and realistically. Mental illness affects people of all age groups, educational backgrounds and financial statuses. There are a number of causes for mental illness, including hereditary, biologic, and social factors.

Myth #6: Mentally strong people haven't experienced roller coaster of emotions

Nugget of truth: Mentally strong people have endured and overcome unbelievable hardships. If they fail in their attempt, they treat their experience as opportunities and become stronger.

Mentally strong people don't use their adversities as an excuse. They're courageous and hold their composure during crisis. When they are stuck, they do ask for help, consult experts and overcome the problem.

Myth #7: Most people suffering from mental illness live in mental hospitals:

Nugget of truth: More than 60% of Americans having mental health problems breathe in their own communities, leading constructive lives. If there is a necessity of hospitalization, they are admitted only for a short time for treatment, and then they are back home. They're no different from people hospitalized for other health problems. A person with a mental illness can recover completely through necessary treatment in hospital.

There are people with a mental illness however, who become homeless, and can benefit from treatment and support in a hospital.

Another myth associated with this is that people with mental health problems think, "If I seek medical assistance for my condition, others might think I'm mad." Don't delay treatment, if it is not getting better.

Reshape Your Mind: 7 Healthy Foods to Take in to Reshape It

Reshaping or building your brain is as important as reshaping your body. Our brain needs quality food to run efficiently. Our memory, concentration, and mood are improved by having an appropriate diet. The brain weighs just about 3 pounds but uses 20% of our calorie intake daily. Our brains need various nutrients for various functions: carbohydrate for power, proteins for the formation of chemicals that the brain needs, and fats to develop healthy brain cells. These foods also contain the nutrients like vitamins, minerals, antioxidants and phytonutrients, necessary to create new brain cells, and safeguard and repair existing cells. The health & vitality of your brain equals a strong memory. Our brain possesses the ability to adapt and change at any age called neuroplasticity. Here are the seven foods particularly essential to building your brain:

- Fruits & Vegetables: contain antioxidants
- Pumpkin Seeds: A handful of these are packed with essential nutrients such as proteins, vitamins, fiber, and minerals.
- Eggs: high in cholesterol and essential fatty acids.
- Avocados: high in Vitamin E, Potassium, and Magnesium.
- Whole Grains: contain fibers, vitamins, and minerals that give a steady stream of energy to the brain.
- Green Tea: helps resist mental fatigue.
- Dark Chocolate: accelerates blood flow to the brain, and boosts concentration.

What Celebrities Say About Mental Illness?

Mental health issues can be worrisome, and make you feel isolated. Public discussion about that subject can prevent that feeling from becoming worse instead of keeping it a secret. According to the National Institute of Mental Illness, about 20% of teens in the age group of 13 to 18 are affected by mental illness.

Here are some open and true stories shared by celebrities about how they dealt with mental health problems:

Justin Bieber

Justin Bieber talked about depression when he called off all his meetings with his fans in future. He said his meetings with them often leave him exhausted and upset.

He definitely needs a break, because depression is not only a mental disorder, but can be the reason for physical symptoms such as pain and fatigue.

Rowan Blanchard

In 2015, Rowan Blanchard had mentioned on Instagram that she had never experienced ups and downs like this year. She said she sometimes had multiple emotions simultaneously, and finally said the ups and downs, and the resulting depression can be put in perspective if they appear too much.

She added, "I learned that everything is temporary, and happiness and sadness can stay within me at the same time."

She said, "The learnings and realizations have helped me understand, enduring and fighting these emotions is better than ostracizing them.

Halsey

In an interview with *Billboard* recently, Halsey, one of the America's busiest new pop singers had mentioned about her battle with mental illness, and her thoughts of committing suicide when she was only 17.

She went on with *Elle* in a quest of eliminating the misconceptions many folks have about mental illness. She said, "Being a bipolar, biracial, and bisexual woman makes me inconvenient at times."

"I'm glad I've sighted a community on the web where I can express my emotions and talk to people alike," she added.

Cara Delevingne

Beautiful and successful people are not immune to depression. Cara Delevingne, one of the top models and actresses revealed at the 2015 Women in the world summit about managing depression for years, because of which she felt completely suicidal.

At the summit, she said, "I once reached a point where there was a mental breakdown that made me feel, I want to live no more."

"It became worse when I felt, I was the only woman affected by this disorder," she said. She was more worried because she felt she was fully isolated."

The beautiful model said her suffering from depression didn't diminish when she succeeded as a model, but she began to wear a bold face. Cara is shining now, and she told Rupert Everett that she got there by being open to some of her close friends.

Conclusion
Depression can be dealt with - face it boldly – open up to your close friends.

Chapter IV

Body Types: Ectomorph, Mesomorph, and Endomorph

Human beings are very different from one another, be it personality, abilities, or physiques. Of all these, a person is first distinguished by his or her body type. These variations are mostly because of heredity.

Scientists came up with the theory of body types in the 1940's, which described 3 main human body types: Ectomorph (Ecto), Endomorph (Endo), and Mesomorph (Meso).

Ectomorph body type
People with ectomorph body type are skinny and lightweight, with small joints and lean muscles. Ecto's typically have long thin limbs and small shoulders. Ectomorphs have a speedy metabolism and less fat. They need to put greater effort to gain weight.

Characteristics of an ectomorph
- Thin delicate bone structure
- Flat chest
- Thin body
- Small shoulders
- Low body fat

Endomorph body type
Endomorphs are exactly the opposite to Ectomorphs. They usually appear large with abundant fat accumulation. They are typically short with an hourglass body (curvaceous) with a waist usually larger than the chest.

Characteristics of Endomorphs

- Round body shape
- Abundant fat accumulation
- Short, thick limbs
- Slower metabolism
- Need great effort to lose weight

Mesomorph body type

If you ask people what body type they desire to possess, it'll not be surprising if most people's answer is mesomorph. Mesomorphs have enormous bone structure, great muscles, and an athletic body. They have features of Ectomorphs as well as Endomorphs. Unlike Ecto's, Meso's require less effort to lose weight.

Characteristics of Mesomorphs

- Muscular
- Strong
- Medium sized joints and bones
- Broad shoulders
- Moderate fat

Why is it important to know your body type?

Scientists came up with the concept of body types to predict how people usually respond to the intake of macronutrients. Understanding body types aka Somatype will help you determine the nutrition and training techniques that are right for you.

It is imperative that we know our body type so as to live a comfortable, healthy lifestyle, following the right diet and exercise plan for us.

Body-type Specific Foods

Right foods for ectomorphs

Are you bored of looking at the same skinny bag of bones every morning in the mirror? If so, spending a few more minutes on this article might help you. The principle behind accumulating pounds is quite simple – just take in more calories than your body burns.

Calories are the basic building blocks of your body. Regularly fund your body with more calories for it to grow. So, the word EAT has to become your mantra. That's not to say you drive directly to McDonalds to get 5 dinner boxes, or KFC to get 5 buckets. Your body needs the right sum of macronutrients to become bigger with bulging muscles.

Ectomorphs are typically marked by a fast metabolic rate and an immense carb tolerance. They do best with a significant amount of carbs in their diet.

Be concerned with 3 main macronutrients distributed in this fashion - Carbohydrates (50%), Proteins (30%), and Fat (20%).

Carbohydrates
Carbohydrates are the best friends for an ectomorph. However, all carbs differ from one another. There are two types of carbs, namely, fast releasing carbs, and slow releasing carbs. Fast releasing carbs are the nutrients that are broken down by the body, lickety-split whereas slow releasing carbs are those that are broken down slowly.

The Glycemic Index scale will tell you the rate at which carbs are digested. In other words, food that is high in fiber and nutrients are digested late, and food low in nutrients, mostly processed, are digested soon.

For low and high-carb foods, refer to: Glycemic Index table

Proteins

Protein, the building block of your body is one of the most important macronutrients. People, especially body builders aiming to top up lean mass need to adopt lean sources of protein in their diet. If you consume large quantities of fatty foods, you'll gain a lot of weight, but not muscle.

Examples of lean sources of protein include, fish, chicken, turkey, eggs, lean steak, cottage cheese, and milk.

Fats

If you think all fats are bad, then that's a misconception you hold like many others. The fact is, fats play a crucial role in the body and are responsible for many functions – lubricate body cells, and maintain the soft feel of your skin and hair. Most importantly, fats regulate a muscle-building hormone called testosterone. Freaks seriously intending to build muscles will not succeed without testosterone.

We've just learned how important fats are, now let's also learn the ways of getting them.

If you're thinking of grabbing the nearest bottle of oil, then you can be sure of increasing cholesterol in your body that increases the risk of cardiac related problems. Be concerned only about Omega 3 fatty acids, the important ones being EPA (Eicosapentaenoic acid) and DHA (Docosahexaenoic acid), found in oily fish and seafood, and ALA (alpha-linolenic acid), found in nuts and seeds. Do not cut back on these fatty acids as they not only help your body function, but also offer some health benefits.

A mixture of fatty acids such as oily fish, eggs, nuts and seeds, avocado, and flaxseed oil.

Right foods for Mesomorphs
People with Mesomorph body type have an inborn athletic physique.

Meso's can easily lose weight. It doesn't mean they can eat anything. They have to follow a well-designed diet and fitness plan to prevent fat gain, and to improve the overall health.

People with Mesomorph body type have an inborn athletic physique with strong muscles. Unlike Endo's, Meso's can lose weight easily. But it doesn't mean they can take in anything. Even they have to follow a well-designed diet and fitness plan to maintain an ideal weight and overall health.

Meso's do best on a diet that consists of a mixture of macronutrients such as carbs, proteins, and fats, in the ratio 4:3:3 (carbohydrates-40%, proteins-30%, and fat-30%).

Right foods for Endomorphs
Endo's as you might have known by now have a greater tendency towards a curvaceous body.

Endomorphs have to be concerned with mostly carb foods in the low range of the Glycemic Index Scale. High-carb foods as mentioned earlier, are foods that are broken down slowly by the body.

High fiber foods including, fruits and veggies and whole grains are the best carb foods for people with this body type.

For slow-digesting, high-carb foods, refer to GI Index: Glycemic Index table

Lean proteins

Proteins are another macronutrient essential for Endo's since they are the most satiating among all macronutrients. So, they fill you up at every meal and you'll not crave for foods and snacks between meals, and restrict calorie intake.

Most protein sources are rich in fat and are not favorable to Endo's. So, they have to count on lean protein sources. Live strong with lean protein sources such as lean beef, pork, egg white, skinless chicken and turkey, fish, and soy food.

Summary

Nutrition plays a pivotal role to make your body and all of its systems work properly, and to have an ideal body weight. It helps reduce body fat, provide energy to your body, and assist sleep.

A balanced diet and exercise are very important to lead a healthy life. However, eating healthy food and no exercise may help you have a healthy body. On the other hand, eating unhealthy food and exercising regularly will not make you a bodybuilder.

Consuming more calories than your body burns will automatically make you gain weight. For that matter, you may become obese. Dropping pounds at any age takes a lot of time and effort after that. Preventing being overweight or obese is much easier.

When you're watching TV, your hands are not tied or occupied on something, and your free hands will quickly grab some snacks for munching. You don't really care how healthy they are. Exercising while watching TV is a good idea.

Weight loss presents to you a multitude of benefits:
- No respiratory problems/snoring
- Prevents chronic diseases
- Reduces weight joint pain
- Psychological benefits

Above all, there are various health benefits because of weight loss.

Metabolism refers to a set of chemical reactions that take place in our body that's responsible for releasing energy for cellular processes.

Every organism needs energy to do any task, or for that matter, to live. Without it, they cease to exist. They need energy that they get from food to grow and reproduce.

There are a number of diet plans that assure weight loss, but most of them make you hungry soon causing you to give up dieting. So, it's important to choose a diet plan that makes you feel full while not eating large portions, helps quickly drop pounds, and speeds up metabolism.

Most people have questions like "How much I should weigh?", "How much weight I should lose?", or "What is my ideal body weight?" All these answers can be found in the table under the topic "How much should I weigh?"

Some people are worried that they're gaining weight in spite of dieting. This is either because of not following the diet plan properly or because of diet mistakes. Gaining weight can be prevented by overcoming the diet mistakes.

There are diet plans that help you lose weight and some to gain weight. A considerable population of Americans are underweight with thin long limbs, a flat tummy, and small shoulders. They die for weight gain as people die for weight loss. Some weight gain diet plans can help them.

The diet plan for diabetes patients is a little different. They have to focus on slow-digesting, high-carb intake as much as possible because high-carb foods cause a slow rise in blood sugar levels. The Glycemic Index table lists some of the most common high-carb foods.

Japan is one of the countries that have the least obese people in the world. Their eating habits and the fact that they do more walking are mostly the reasons.

Inspired by great bodybuilders, most people do everything they can to have a gym body, but don't talk much about mental strength. They must realize that building mental strength is as important as building muscles to have a better state of mind. Self-motivation, personal identity, and social identity constitute mental strength.

Shaping the brain needs quality food. Some foods that help build the brain are listed under the topic "Reshaping The Brain."

Mental illness can be really worrisome, and can make you feel alone psychologically. Nearly 20% of teens in America suffer from mental illness. Some top celebrities have shared their episodes of mental illness and how they succeeded in overcoming it.

We know that every person differs from another in personality, abilities, and body type (skinny, athletic, or obese) or Somatype. However, we immediately recognize a person by his or her body type. Technically, there are three body types: Ectomorph, Endomorph, and Mesomorph.

Understanding the body types will help you determine the nutrition and training that fit your body type.

Look for other books by Roman Iver:

5 Secrets on How To Lose Weight And Start Looking and Feeling Great + Effective Weight Loss Recipes

Link: https://www.amazon.com/dp/B01JQML4S4

AND

Diet and Weight Loss Doesn't Have to Be Hard

Link: https://www.amazon.com/dp/B0167ON9W8

www.ingramcontent.com/pod-product-compliance
Lightning Source LLC
Chambersburg PA
CBHW070242290526
45789CB00004B/1726